Our Journey:

Diary of a Caregiver

Our Journey:

Diary of a Caregiver

by
KENNETH VOGT

BEACON HILL PRESS OF KANSAS CITY
Kansas City, Missouri

ISBN: 083-411-433X

Printed in the
United States of America

Cover Design: Crandall Vail

10   9   8   7   6   5   4   3   2   1

In Memory

RUBY C. VOGT

My beautiful and gifted Ruby was stricken by the terrifying and terminal Alzheimer's disease. The autopsy clearly confirmed the earlier diagnosis.

Day by day I watched her brilliant mental powers fade into the shadows, and then it was all darkness. She struggled against that darkness with all her diminished powers until she could do no more. The struggle remains with all of us to find an answer. In this account, I spill out the raw humanness of our journey, not in despair but in hope.

Contents

Preface

These are very personal glimpses of our journey. Alzheimer's is not something that happened to Ruby. It happened to *us*. Alzheimer's was our affliction. In many ways, the more intimate our relationship, the more heart-breaking the journey became.

Ours was a close working-playing relationship. We reared our two sons together, and we worked together in Christian ministry. In many ways we were almost perfectly matched. I was the leader, the preacher, the assertive, aggressive promoter of ideas, and she was the implementer and influencer. In our churches I was the one that got us into trouble, and she was the stiller of the storms.

Introduction

No one knows what causes Alzheimer's disease. It was first identified in 1906 by Alois Alzheimer, a German neurologist. His patient, a 55-year-old woman, was too young to be senile but had similar symptoms. After she died, an autopsy revealed clusters of debris and a strange jumble of tangles in her brain.[1]

In Alzheimer's disease, the degenerated nerve endings in the outer layer of the brain prevent electrochemical signals from passing between cells. The more degeneration, the more devastating the impact on the brain's "executive actions"—memory, emotion, and higher intellectual functioning.[2]

Among the elderly, Alzheimer's disease is the fourth-leading cause of death (after heart disease, cancer, and stroke). In America, 2.5 million are afflicted. Canada adds 300,000 more victims.

Alzheimer's strips its victims of their physical skills, their sanity, and their self-esteem. The mind goes first, then the body, until the victim is reduced to a helpless zombie. But until a person reaches that point, he is plagued by a kaleidoscope of frightening emotions. The process, usually stretching over years, is agonizing.[3]

I can look back now and see signs of the disease some eight years before Ruby's death. She took some women home from a church meeting and arrived at her own house much later than usual. "I got lost!" she exclaimed.

The warning sign, though, that really jolted me was when she could no longer balance our checkbook. She always had delighted in doing it, but suddenly two and two just didn't make four. That really hit me. What lay ahead would be infinitely worse than I had ever imagined. Journey's end would come after a long and torturous descent into pain, misery, and grief. God's grace sustained as we walked that road together.

· 1 ·

Family Times

Living with an Alzheimer's victim certainly isn't dull. Every day offers a new surprise and challenge. We exist in a twilight zone of lucidity interspersed with irrationality. Yesterday, I prepared to leave her for an hour to run a necessary errand. Carefully, I explained the situation to her and provided for her every need. Apparently, a few moments after I left, she felt her "father-mother" had deserted her. Terrified, she fled to the neighbors.

I thank God for His providence that put us in Sequestra, a caring Christian retirement community of 31 units, envisioned by the sainted Roger Taylor 10 years ago. How good it is to feel the comfort and understanding of this extended family and a nearby caring church and good pastor!

Anniversary Anguish

I planned a special 46th wedding anniversary breakfast for just the two of us. The children sent greeting cards.

The cards didn't seem to help her very much, but they helped me mightily. We also received a beautiful gold, embossed card from the prime minister of Canada, one from the premier of British Columbia, and even one from the queen of England. Instead of going to breakfast, I drove her around the countryside to give her some quietness and peace. It was a troubling time.

Losing Identity

Upon arriving at church, she would ask me, "How shall I introduce you?" I would say, "Well, who am I?" She would reply, "My father." After a while I went along with the game, confident that people would understand.

How I thank God for my own health! It allows me to care for her and help her struggle with the jigsaw puzzle. I rejoice in every piece that fits, though the puzzle is never completed.

Growing Backward

With Alzheimer's, life is unreeled backward through teen years, puberty, childhood, and finally the comfortable world of the mother's womb—comfortable, that is, except for the mother. That is what I am becoming now. After a while, my "child" will tear from the mother's womb into the eternal.

These are some of my deep, private thoughts when Ruby's illness overwhelms me. Alzheimer's is a stealthy, silent stealer. Daily, sometimes hourly, it takes the beautiful Ruby that I have known for all these 46 years of ministry. She is stolen away by bits and pieces. What is left is a body without a brain. The rationality that makes a being human is gone. Her conclusions, reached emotionally, are totally foreign to our human experiences.

· 2 ·

Years of Joy

The years of joy, of intimate conversations, of discussing problems, of conferring on decisions, have ended. In some ways, she is a child—resentful, rebellious, exasperating—but a child impossible to correct or discipline. A child is always disciplined in hope of improvement. But in this case no such hope exists.

Separation Without a Termination

Society accustoms us to think of death as a separation with a fixed terminus. A memorial service is conducted. Grief is vented and healed through the presence of friends, the hymns of the Church, and the caring love of a minister. In our case, death has already taken place without the benefit and release of a memorial service. The Ruby that I once knew is gone!

Even the birth of our two sons, now strong, fine family men, is only a hazy recollection to her. She is living now in her adolescent years before our marriage. She cannot recall our beautiful and simple wedding ceremony at 8 A.M. on a Sunday morning in her home church.

Forgiveness

She may put on her day clothes at night and go to bed. When I try to correct her, she is sure she is right. Sometimes I let it be. Sometimes I remonstrate with her. Some-

15

times I change her, but then she tends to be very frustrated with herself and resentful toward me.

Often she asks me to forgive her. Always I say, "Yes." Sometimes I hug her and assure her of my forgiveness, though she does not really need it. She is not guilty nor responsible for her actions. Her brain is eroded and simply does not work. Yet at times, she is naughty like a child and knows it. In those times, forgiveness is real.

· 3 ·

The Strangling Net

Daily, the net is strangling the sanity out of my Ruby. Brief moments of near lucidity come, followed immediately by the far-off yesterday again. Before the Lord, I feel we are being ground to powder. Where is our life together? Even mercy escapes us. There is nothing but the black shadow of increasing despair.

Evil Being

Evil voices and people suggest impure actions to her. She resists them with all her might because she is a pure woman. We have been faithful to each other for a lifetime, with no desire for clandestine and illicit relationships. Yet she thinks of herself as an evil woman. Often in her good years, as I observed her face in the congregation, I would see in her the reflection of God.

Force of Habit

She can still pray a beautiful prayer of thanksgiving at the dinner table. She can lead an opening prayer in the midst of the congregation at the beginning of a worship service.

Understanding

I am beginning to discern and understand when she is slipping away more deeply. I can sense her observing me—

wondering who I am. She will begin with questions, trying to pinpoint my identity. "What is your first name? Are you the Kenneth who lived in Meade, Kans.? Did you have brothers and sisters? What are their names?" and on and on. "Are you that other Kenneth?"

The Locket Watch

I gave her a heart-shaped locket watch inscribed with her name and phone number. That was a total mystery to her. She said, "People will look at this when I get lost and know who I am." I finally shortened the chain so that she could not get it off. Then she would force it open and hide it. When she was wearing it, she would always say her father gave it to her.

Firmness

I tried being firm with her. When she insisted on an impossible course of action, I forcefully contradicted her. It hurt me to do that, for we have never spoken to each other like that. At the moment, the reproof seemed to get through. After a while she said, "Some man spoke very harshly to me a while ago." I felt like a heel. She also questions my Christianity. Says she, "If you were a Christian, you would understand and let me do what I want to do."

Most Baffling Times

The most baffling times of all are those when she does not know me. She mixes me into that unseen, evil world around her. As far as I know, there never were any men in her life who threatened her or abused her in any way. And yet that surfaces into her mind. When those times occur, I am the helpless outsider. I can only try to provide a caring person in my stead.

Sweet Release

In dark night hours, I can think of death as a sweet

release. My own death, however, would make her the responsibility of her sons, and her care would come from strangers. That responsibility they should not have to assume. My responsibility is unending. Our commitment to each other was "for better—for worse, for richer—for poorer, in sickness and in health, to love and to cherish, till death us do part." I would never repudiate that promise.

At the same time, death would be a sweet release for her and for me. Her mansions are ready. Her faith in a living Savior remained strong and unwavering from her childhood. From her conversion at the age of five, she has wanted nothing contrary to the will of God. Now Alzheimer's has stolen her capacity for faith. Faith and trust are capacities of the mind. When disease shrivels the mind, faith and trust have no place of residence.

So it is a body without a mind. We have prayed for healing. We have been anointed and prayed for by the spiritual leaders of the church. We are walking in faith now, but the waiting process is so long—so very long.

Conversation

Sometimes she asks me why we don't converse like we once did. How does one converse with an irrational partner? Baby talk might be appropriate, but how do you do that with an adult?

She speaks to me about events that happen only in the deep recesses of her own mind and wonders why I don't know about them. She wonders why I don't see the same people in the room that she sees. When I assure her that only the two of us are here, she looks at me as if to say, "Now you are deceiving me."

• 4 •

Sustaining Life

Why does our Christian society insist that we must sustain the body's life after mind has flown? To raise the question is startling. I don't know the answer for society—or for myself. What really is life? Is not human life body, soul, and spirit? When the body dies, it takes the mind with it, and the spirit returns to God. When the mind dies, what do we do with the body? Should we not let it go too? At least, not prevent it from going? Should we assist it? God be merciful to us in our dilemma.

Prayer

O God, through our Lord Jesus Christ, I come to You. You are the Sovereign of the universe, but You also know where we are. You know our human condition. You know the pain and anguish I felt this morning as I left Ruby for this overnight trip. She thinks I need to make this trip in order to attend a district preacher's meeting because I am now an interim pastor on the Washington Pacific District. The truth is, I need this trip to preserve my own health and sanity. Ray and Lorene Finger from Alaska are staying with her. They are longtime friends. Lorene is such a caring, outgoing person; I couldn't ask for a better helper. I praise You for her. Amen.

It Is Tough

Ruby clung to me and cried. She could not seem to understand that Ray and Lorene were longtime friends and staying with her. She was terribly afraid. She said, "They will come and kill me." No one knows who "they" are. "They" are dragons created by her own imagination.

Twisted

The devastating effects of this illness sometimes makes "they" become me. "They" become men who help her dress and shower. That is me. I am that person—lovingly, tenderly, and carefully arranging her clothes and helping her into them. Logical sequencing has completely left her. She may put on a bra over her blouse or try to put on pantyhose over her slacks.

Deviousness

There is a deviousness that goes with this illness also. Sometimes she clings to me, as she did this morning. At other times she slyly lets me know that it would be all right for me to leave—perhaps for good. She was a beautiful companion, helpmate, career partner, and wife and mother for 40 years. I owe her my life for the rest of her time. I pray God for health to outlive her so that I can care for her. This is more than duty; it is the service of love. No rejection on her part will ever turn me away. I know her true self. We belong to each other for life.

Keep a Diary

Yesterday, one of our social workers told me to keep a diary. I had started one some weeks ago, not sure that I should. It is very personal and intimate. She said, "Do it for your own sake and for your children. Afterward they need to know about your journey together."

· 5 ·

Loving Care

I often thank God that we are in Sequestra among a caring Christian community—and in Canada. That, too, is the providence of God. We never consciously planned that. It just sort of happened. God led us here—no doubt about it. We are in the will of God.

This is true for many reasons, not the least of which is Canadian health care—all doctors' visits, medicines, hospital stays, and daily home care is available at minimal cost. The sophisticated testing devices at the University of British Columbia Research Center are part of the provincial plan. For this we pay $220 twice a year. Of course, it is not without benefit to British Columbia. We brought our stateside money here and built a house here. We pay taxes, too, but they are very reasonable. And, of course, I was born here and hold my Canadian citizenship with pride.

The Professionals

Without exception, the professionals who are helping us have demonstrated incredible compassion. This is true of doctors, researchers, social workers, and nurses. The patience of nurses who cope with Ruby's wandering around and trying to help is remarkable. One day she was helping the nurse push her service cart. Ruby was draped in a faded hospital robe and was wearing long white stockings that had slipped down around her ankles. She looked like a scarecrow. When I remonstrated with them about the arrangement, the nurse said, "Oh, that is all right, Ruby is helping me." *Wow!*

Trying Harsh Words

We visited our son Randy and his family in Nebraska. On the way home, when Ruby went into an uncontrollable, crying, pleading, praying mood, begging me to take her home, I tried harshness. I commanded her to stop. She did for a short time. Then she plaintively said, "A while ago some man spoke very harshly to me, and I am scared." I assured her we were going home, that home was west, but it did no good. In her mind, her home was in western Kansas with her parents. What awful tricks this disease plays with the mind. Her behavior is childish. Her responses are erratic and unpredictable. This condition does not respond to discipline.

Supportive Prayer Group

Yesterday, I took Ruby to the ladies' Bible study and prayer group here at Sequestra. The men began meeting again, too, as we do in the fall and winter months. I heard Arnold pray for Ruby. How good it was to feel his compassionate understanding. He prayed, "Lord, we cannot understand. We can only trust, and sometimes it is hard to do that. Can this thing that is happening to us, contrary to all our hopes and dreams, be the will of God? If this is Your will, then bend us to it."

· 6 ·

What We Want and What We Get

Both of us have wanted nothing but the will of God in all our mature years, and we have done the will of God. It is not self-righteous or egocentric to say that. It is simply true. Then the question comes: "What are You doing with us now? What more do You want?" We can only believe the scripture that says God is always making a purpose out of everything, good and bad (Rom. 8:28). He has a divine intentionality that transcends our knowledge and springs out of His eternal, unending love. With Job, we must say, "Though he slay me, yet will I trust in him" (13:15). Without this deep-rooted confidence what is there? At best, nothingness. At worst, bitterness.

No Fairness or Justice

The other day, I described to Ruby's doctor the kind of life Ruby had lived. She never tasted wine or liquor. She never smoked a cigarette. She has been free from all medications. Rarely did she take aspirin. She has been a wonderful wife, mother, and helpmate. She lived by high ideals. And now this! The doctor is helpless in the face of our dilemma, and she said, "It just isn't fair." She cannot change our condition, but it does help to feel her empathy.

24

Losing Her Without
Saying Good-bye

Alzheimer's disease is a monstrous thing. It is worse than death. It silently, inexorably steals our loved ones away. It takes them into the void of nothingness without giving us the benefit of saying good-bye and experiencing the healing of a memorial service. It is a death without a burial. When physical death finally comes, it is hard to grieve properly. There is no other monster like this in the world.

Giving Care in Deep Grief

The caregiver must now serve 24 hours a day in the deep throes of grief. Friends and loved ones are not permitted to speak caring words of comfort. That would be presumptuous, for there is still a body to be dealt with and cared for. Could not our advanced society find a better way? Must we still be governed by ancient laws related to death? Must caregivers preserve at all costs a physical body when this living death has robbed life of all that is meaningful when memory is gone? When all rational thought has gone? When emotions are so entangled that they make no sense? When a gentle kiss may be interpreted as an attempted rape?

Sex

We had a good sex life. Both of us were passionate but restrained. Sexual union was a constant wonder and delight, not a right demanded but a privilege granted.

As Ruby's disease continued, she became more amorous. It was as if she was desperately clutching a relationship that she sensed was slipping away.

However, it wasn't long until something new and startling entered the relationship. She whispered to me one day, "Honey, I think I am going to have a baby." I laughed, and that was a mistake. She was hurt that I would not believe her announcement. I tried to explain to her that old people don't have babies, but that did not help. She was living in premarriage years, and the thought of having a baby filled her with terrifying guilt. Premarital sex was forbidden by Christian ideals that we both shared deeply.

After this, our whole relationship was altered. To caress her aroused suspicion and fear. I had to change my ways of showing her my love, and love became even more meaningful.

· 7 ·

Reaching for a Miracle

The cause and cure of Alzheimer's disease eludes medical science. Our sophisticated and expensive testing devices leave us with a modicum of uncertainty. Is it really this illness? Are the symptoms indicative of other reversible forms of dementia? So we go into the never-never land of diagnosis by rule-out of all other causes. It is slow, tedious, and uncertain.

The caregiver is easy prey to anything that promises a cure or even a relief. I confess that I listen to the subtle promises. When medical science has nothing to offer, then experimentation is better than nothing. Such an attitude may not be wise, but this is what the caregiver thinks, feels, and sometimes admits.

There is always the possibility of a divine miracle. I believe in that too. I have witnessed some miraculous results in answer to the prayer of faith. But I have also stood at many gravesides; some were short and some longer. Death is no respecter of age.

Whether a physical miracle comes or not, there is the miracle of a God-given peace in the midst of dark despair. I have experienced that.

Without faith in the Supreme Being who is always working to make good out of bad, my life would be hopeless indeed. Health, goodwill, righteousness, and peace ultimately will win. It may take all of this world and a part of

27

the next to bring the triumph to pass. The ancient saw it when he wrote, "The earth shall be filled with the knowledge of the glory of the Lord, as the waters cover the sea" (Hab. 2:14).

The Waiting List

The thought of going on a waiting list for institutionalized care shakes me to my toes. Her doctor and the social worker both advised me to do that right away. The implications of that are only sinking in several days later. Does it really have to come to that? Sober reflection convinces me I ought to prepare for that, but I shrink from the first step. It may be a year before her name would come to the top. There are legal considerations. My Ruby needs to give me the power of attorney while she is able to do so without her competence being questioned. There are financial considerations. While we are not wealthy, we do have some options. There are caregivers who have nothing but bleak desolation at the point of their finances. Medicare in the States generally has no provision for long-term institutional care. Those in the Canadian health care system have a different set of hoops to negotiate.

I retreat from the terrible responsibility of taking that first step toward the waiting list. Reason and experience both tell us that we are on a long, downward spiral. Just the thought of that final placement into an institution has kept me from making those first inquiries. Yet I know it must be done. To delay any longer would be foolish, and so I yield to the advice of doctor and social worker. These people must surely know better than I do, even though my heart says, "No, no!"

I would like to try a live-in housekeeper person. Our home permits that arrangement. The housekeeper would have private quarters. So that is our first alternative. Just the same, I must take the step of getting her onto a waiting list. Tomorrow? . . . tomorrow? . . . tomorrow. I really must do that one day next week.

Hopelessness in Their Eyes

Hopelessness is especially observable in those who are working on this disease from the medical side. Presently, they have nothing to offer except sedatives. They give medication to alleviate stress. They give sleeping potions of one kind or another. Sometimes they try antidepressant medication. That might be good for me! With each remedy they try, they are careful to ask what the effects are, for they do not know. This is not to put them down. I appreciate the mystery they face and their dedicated quest for an answer.

This hopelessness is not so observant in the social workers. These people work to make Alzheimer's bearable, especially to the caregiver, so they give hopeful suggestions from time to time. These include turning mirrors to the wall so that victims will not attach reality to images.

I have found that television is seldom helpful, regardless of the type of programming. It populates her world with imaginary folks who are real to her. At her present state of regression, these folks are all evil, whether men or women, sometimes even children. And they do evil, vulgar things. As far as we know, she never has been molested and has lived a sheltered life. Where do these evil thoughts come from?

The Greatest Shock up to Now

One day, it dawned on me she was lumping me into that evil world. In my poor human way of reasoning, there is no basis for that. Those who knew us best through the years knew we were kind, thoughtful, and considerate.

We had disagreements, of course. In fact, one of the great contributions Ruby made to our partnership was her willingness to disagree with ideas and suggestions I proposed. She tested them with the strength of her own will. Sometimes she changed my mind to the good. When we had been through one of these critique sessions, I always felt the plan we were operating on was better than the one I had originally proposed. Our history proves that to be true. But now, suddenly I realized she was putting me in that evil world about her. I became a part of "they" and "them." For the moment, she had lost who I was. Then how do I help and comfort?

· 8 ·

Powerless to Help

For the first time, I encountered despair. How could I help when she saw my efforts coming out of that evil empire around her? She attributed my kindest suggestions to evil intentions. The subtlety of the human mind in this condition is almost beyond comprehension. The other day during our prayer time at her bedside, she suddenly said, "You make me very uncomfortable." That was a shock. We had enjoyed all the other evenings. She had participated and prayed some beautiful prayers. God seemed very real. How wonderful to sense her beautiful spirit coming through to commune with the Divine Maker. I prayed and mentioned the beauties of heaven and the glories of the world. She immediately misinterpreted that and said, "It sounds like you are planning to take me out and bury me."

Logical Sequencing Is Lost

Loss of logical sequencing was an early and major consequence of Ruby's disease. She could not move from one logical process to its successor. The brain simply skips to something else entirely unrelated. This is now happening also in her language structure. She will start a sentence, moving in one direction of thought; and then, without a break, she will speak about the next object her eyes see. She starts talking about making the bed and then shifts to a book lying on the stand.

31

During our early years in the ministry, when fabrics were not what they are today, she took great pride in the appearance of my shirts. She still beautifully irons my shirts. However, I must make sure she has the iron in her hand. The other day she called down to me in my office-study, saying, "This thing won't work." When I came up, she was trying to iron my shirt with the electric teakettle.

It Is So Dark

For a while Ruby was hospitalized. "It is so dark," Ruby told me last night as I sat by her bedside in the hospital. "It is so dark." The darkness was filled with imaginary evil people she could not identify and with sneering and taunting voices. She was terror-stricken to the very core of her being. In such moments, she tries to run away or contemplates suicide. What torment this must be, and it torments me to see her in this condition. My lovely, thoughtful, compassionate Ruby devastated by this onslaught of wickedness. With the Psalmist David, I cry out, "Oh, where are You? Why do You not answer me?"

Forks, Knives, and Spoons

Many times forks, knives, and spoons are all the same to her, although she feeds herself very well. The other day I had set out our TV trays and placed the food there. We sat down and said our table grace; then I realized we did not have forks. Since she was closest to the kitchen, I said, "Honey, would you get us a couple of forks, please?" Instead of forks she brought knives. When I told her we needed forks, she went back and got more knives. At this point, she realized what she was doing and had an awful sense of frustration and inadequacy. That is tough.

Take Me Home

Today she begged me to take her home. How do you handle that when you *are* home? We have talked about

32

home. Where is home? We have talked about her parents. She may remember they have gone to heaven long ago. We have talked about the deed to this house and how we bought it with our own money. Her name is on the deed, and I have shown her that. "This is our house—our home. See these pictures on the wall? These are our sons and their families." In the next breath, she begs me to take her home. Other times I simply say, "OK, let's go." We go out for a ride, ending back here at our house, and for a little while it may be home.

Why Didn't You Tell Me!

She often chides me for not telling her in advance of going to church, the store, or wherever. We may have talked about an event for days or weeks and written it on calendars. We did that with our Christmas trip to our eldest son's house. We prepared packages to take with us. She helped as she could to wrap them. When the morning came to go and we were getting ready, she accused me of just ordering her around without telling her of our plans.

No Money

For quite some time she didn't want to carry any money, but I insisted she ought to have some change and bills. She could not be trusted with larger amounts. Of late, she has been asking for more money. I think in her mind she is planning a trip home. If she had all the money in the world, it would be utterly impossible for her to travel alone. She couldn't get to the end of the first block. She doesn't know her own house address or telephone number.

Save the Mother

Society has largely accepted the idea that the mother must be saved even at the price of the unborn infant. What happens in Alzheimer's disease is that the patient regresses day after day into the womb of society, causing an intolerable burden. To help such patients, society and the medical world are diminishing the care and attention they should be giving to those whose afflictions are reversible, those who have hope of quality life. Somehow attention must be focused on preserving the whole person and not just the physical aspects.

Where Is the Line?

When has the Alzheimer's victim regressed into the womb of society until all hope is gone? Will we continue to sacrifice the life of the caregiver to the point of complete exhaustion and even death itself? There are many instances where the caregiver dies before the victim. Is that the preservation of life according to the high standard of the Judeo-Christian ethic? We now tend to back away from that hard question. I whisper it only now to my intimate tape recorder and say it is God's business. We do not do that in the case of the mother and the unborn child. We make a decision. Why should we not make a decision in the case of an Alzheimer's victim who has regressed without hope of any significant life? Oh, perish the thought.

Please Eat, Please Eat

The request "Please eat" was said to an old woman in the next hospital bed by her young granddaughter. It was shrieked into her ear because she was obviously deaf. She is also an Alzheimer's victim. By refusing to eat, her body was saying, "Let me die. My time is over." But the granddaughter was begging her to eat. We have to ask, to what purpose? Why do we make such desperate effort to prolong life after all sense of reality is lost?

The "Thank You" Is Gone

In our home "Thank you" was a very frequent phrase. We said, "Thank you," to God at the table grace and often to each other through the day. Our boys also picked up that act of courtesy and used it easily. When they didn't, we reminded them. Now "Thank you" is no longer in Ruby's vocabulary or, as far as I can tell, in her emotions. Whatever I do for her is simply accepted as a matter of course. A small child doesn't say, "Thank you," either, except when coaxed. Ruby has regressed to a small-child stage in most circumstances. She may still say, "Thank you," to others who do some good deed for her, but not to me.

Squeaky Doors

All my life, I have been oiling squeaky doors. It became a point of humor with pastors under my jurisdiction. If I found squeaky doors in churches, I would laughingly remind them it was a part of their job to stop the squeak. Now I am thankful for squeaky doors. That is how life changes. They alert me that Ruby is moving stealthily about the house. She is trying to escape from some of these "people" that inhabit her world. To her, the house is frequently full of people. At first they were mostly men. In the course of weeks, she included women. Of late, her fears have been from children. She may wake me in the middle of the night and urge me to take care of the children. She never talks about *our* children. It is always *the* children. In her mind, we are not married.

Very Lost

Yesterday she was disoriented, and it continued this morning. I thought it might help her if she could talk long-distance to her sister, so I gave the phone receiver to her. As she began to talk to her sister, she said, "There is some strange man here in my house trying to help me make this telephone call." That startled her sister, so I had to come on the line to tell her that strange man was only me!

I Shudder to Think

I shudder to think how difficult it would be if our roles

were reversed, and I was the victim and she the caregiver. All our lives I was the leader, the decision maker, and she was the influencer and implementer. She beautifully carried out the course of action. Now I must take both roles. Suppose she was called on now to direct my life. The situation would be intolerable for her and for me. Many couples have faced role reversals. Husbands who have been the principal car drivers all their lives must surrender that right. It is traumatic. Keys have to be hidden, and time for travel brings a clash of wills. If we look around a bit, we can always find someone whose condition is worse than ours. I wouldn't trade my cross for some I see other people carrying.

"Honey, Don't Hound Me!"

I make a confession now. I spoke those words in a sharp tone of voice. It surprised me. I felt bad about it, for we had never spoken to each other harshly. It showed me how close to a breaking point I really am. She had pestered me for a couple of hours with unanswerable questions. "Please take me home. What are we doing here anyway, since we are not married? Who are you? What is your first name? If we are going to live together in this house, we at least ought to be married." Over and over again, we go down forgotten memory lanes. We look at wedding pictures. We talk about friends who stood up with us and about her beloved pastor. The pastor's daughter was her closest friend and still is to this day. All of this to no avail. Finally I said those sharp words, and it hurt her. I can see her now as she turned and walked away, without tears. She just walked away.

She Ignores My Pain

For about three months I have had a pain in my left shoulder and arm. I sought medical help. It doesn't seem to be anything dangerous, and so I'm living with it. It would help me if she realized I was coping, but she doesn't. As she regresses into childhood, she becomes increasingly dominated by her own world. This beautiful, unselfish person to whom friends would rally because she cared so much is leaving it all up to me to carry on our contact with friends. So I have organized our Christmas card list—our "Christmas family"—of some 300 persons. She has no interest in that, although she still reads with me the cards and letters that come in response.

Kind Neighbors

This Christmas season the neighbors in this immediate Sequestra community have been so kind, bringing us many personally baked Christmas sweets. They know I don't bake much. At the moment of receiving those goodies she is responsive, but in a few minutes she has forgotten who brought them. So "thank-you" notes are my business too.

Hope and Despair

Every day, a caregiver could alternate between hope and despair if he allows those emotions to peak because of some action the Alzheimer's victim engaged in. It is a constantly changing world. At first in the good moments I would think that perhaps Ruby was experiencing a miraculous healing, only to be dashed on the rocks of despair before the day was out by some other deteriorating action. So I am learning to keep life on an even keel. I neither give up hope nor allow myself to be swallowed by despair.

Enjoy the Good Moments

Every cognitive observation is welcomed and enjoyed, like the coming of the birds to the feeder or the abundance of the Christmas tree lights noticed. There is a beauty of a cloud formation with the silver lining at sunset. There is much good mixed with bad when we look for it.

• 9 •

The Living Death Continues

Physical death is not the worst that can happen to people. This death of the mind called Alzheimer's disease sets this disease apart from all others. It reduces life to a great emptiness.

When physical death occurs, one's grief can be allayed by friends and loved ones and a memorial service. But with Alzheimer's, the memory ties are gone. Conversation is a constant effort to reach out to something that isn't there. To attempt to inject memory pieces into such a mind often accentuates the consciousness of the loss. It tends to raise the level of frustration for the victim. So we scoot around in the shallow moments of what is immediately at hand, and conversation goes something like this: "It is time to get dressed now. Here, you have to put this piece on first. Come, take your medication. Here is your purse, honey."

The Other Night

I was not restless, but very wakeful, for long hours of the night, so I stretched out on the divan in the front room to lie and think and read some. After a while, she came out of the bedroom and, like an apparition, moved silently in the dim light. Slowly, tentatively, she moved about from place to place. I tried to imagine what was going on in her mind. I don't think she knew where she was, for she made no recognition of the fact I was there. She had an afghan in her hand and began to spread it out in front of the fireplace. It was sad to see her vain attempts to make a pallet on which to rest. She worked at it for at least half an hour, like a little puppy struggling around in a box, trying to be comfortable. After a while, my heart ached for her so much I couldn't stand it. I said to her, "Honey, would you like me to make you some hot chocolate?" Without registering any surprise at my voice or any remembrance of what she had been doing, she said, "I think that might be nice."

Churchgoing

I'm concerned about churchgoing tomorrow. Last Sunday, Ruby became restless, and we had to leave. We left several times, intending to come back, but it didn't work. In the evening, I was the guest speaker, and she sat with a dear friend. The friend told me later she became restless again, and they did slip out several times. One of the remarks she made to her friend was, "When will that man up there ever get through?" Truthfully, I spoke only 35 minutes, and the whole service was only 65 minutes long.

So, now we face the challenge of what to do on Sunday. During the week, I tried to take her to a Billy Graham film. That didn't work at all. She couldn't endure it, so we came home. If this continues, it will certainly make a change in our life-style. Churchgoing has been a habit of ours since before we were married, and we have gone together now for over 46 years. We were married in church. We dedicated our sons in church. Many of life's great moments have happened to us in the sanctuary. So now what? We'll see how it goes tomorrow.

No Noon, No Night

We are so committed to seasons, years, months, weeks, days, and hours—even seconds. Our sleeping and waking are controlled by segments of time. But the Alzheimer's victim has no such sense of time. Just as we had finished a good lunch and had cleaned up the dishes, she asked when we would eat today. The good ladies who take care of Ruby at day care amuse me a bit. They are very careful to have me tell her when I will return to pick her up. Little do they know that time means nothing to her. When I pick her up, she may not have missed me or may wonder why I was gone so long. She can leave her watch for days and not miss it, then suddenly become almost frantic: "Where is my watch, where, where?" Fortunately as a good caregiver, I remember exactly where I put it. The fact is, I hid it, for she was always losing it. Had I not done that, no one would know where it is. She hides things often. Even darkness and light seem to make little difference. Her eyes are perfectly functional, but her mind does not tell her the difference. I have to put night-lights at strategic places. They are not sufficient to read by, but she will come out of her bedroom and announce she has been reading.

No Shock

For a while, I was at the stage in my care giving that I thought nothing could shock me anymore about this strange affliction. Then it dawned on me that getting into bed was an increasingly difficult procedure for her. I had erroneously assumed you simply got into bed and lay down. But not so. To understand this phenomenon, I have watched her many minutes at a time. Sometimes, she gets so frustrated with this complicated problem of getting into bed that she will just go away and give it up entirely for the time being. I'm still amazed at its complexity.

Now I have had to learn how to get her into bed. At the moment, the easiest way is for her to sit down well back on the bed, and then I simply turn her whole body. I will fluff her pillow under her head, and she may hold her head off the pillow for long moments until I gently press her forehead downward. Then I help her straighten her legs and tuck the blanket under her chin. Then I whisper into her ear words of love and sing a chorus and say a prayer. Sometimes at this stage she may say, "I love you too." How my heart aches for her—and for me, when I'm honest with myself.

There Is Somebody in There

Can you imagine living in your own home and constantly thinking other people are in the house? I would direct her toward the bathroom door. She will come back to me and say, "I can't go in because there is someone there." I can't imagine the complexity of her world. We like to think that diminished powers of intellect simplify her world. The opposite is true. Her world is immensely complex, complicated, and out of control. This is one argument for institutional care. Good institutional care for Alzheimer's victims reduces life to its barest simplicity, where there is only one room. I can see some value in that.

Out to Tea

At the present time Ruby and I go out to tea once or twice a week. A whole host of couples have volunteered that. They want to help us, and I'm so grateful. I'm not at all sure it helps Ruby, but I know it helps me. Their caring and willingness and compassion is such a ministry. They are giving me far more than they know. Without such caring I think I would want to die. In fact, I would gladly die if that would make Ruby better. That is not the way life is. I am dying by inches to give Ruby the care and comfort she must have. My prayer is that I shall outlive her. How much of life is left after that is rather immaterial to me now.

41

· 10 ·

Treasuring the Highlights

The other evening, after I had tucked Ruby into bed as you would a little child, I knelt by her bedside for prayer. Then I said to her, "Why don't we turn on a musical piece before we pray." I pushed the button, and in a little bit I heard Ruby singing along in a clear alto voice, "Learning to lean, learning to lean, / Learning to lean on Jesus," and she never missed a word. That was a comfort to my heart then and is a treasure in my thoughts now. We need to coach ourselves to capture and hold the highlights.

Honey, I Love You

The words "Honey, I love you" are often in my vocabulary as I tenderly touch her, but rarely does she say anything in return. The Ruby that I have known is gone. This dreadful disease stole her away. However, in the stillness of one night, she whispered across to me, "Honey, I love you." What a highlight that was and is.

We know human love is not everything. God's love is infinitely greater. But human love is still the most meaningful of all human emotions. How good it is to know that this disease has not yet robbed her of the desire and ability to express human love.

As an Angel Sent from God

Years ago a lady by the name of Irene Tremer was in one of our churches on the Sacramento District. Because I was the district leader, she knew us better than we knew her. We had not heard of her for about 12 years. Through mutual friends she learned about our plight. As she tells it, "God told me to come help you take care of Ruby." So she came. We met her at the Bellingham airport a week ago last Tuesday. Truly her coming is ordained of God.

She and Ruby get along well. Ruby enjoys Irene, though at times Irene has to be firm with her. Yesterday when I came in, they were seated side by side on the divan, and Irene was fixing Ruby's fingernails. The look of pleasure on Ruby's face was enough to tell me she was enjoying this closeness. What a lifesaver for me.

Ministries

In keeping with my belief that God is always bringing something good out of bad, doors are opening to me for various ministries. I spoke to the nursing association, and as near as I could tell, the leaders wanted me to generate a renewal of compassion in the hearts of the nurses. Nursing, like much else we do in the caring professions, can become mechanical. When that happens to a nurse, she has lost her greatest healing asset.

I did this by showing a large picture of Ruby taken a few years ago. She was a beautiful, caring, gentle person. Then I described to them her present helpless condition. Their hearts were touched, and some tears flowed. The well of compassion was refreshed. Along with that, I was able to express my profound gratitude for the many kindnesses shown us. It was a good meeting.

I spoke also to the hospice society and showed them the documentary done about Ruby by KCVU (Channel 13) and the University of B.C. Research Center. They taught me much more than I could teach them. These volunteers are devoted to making death a meaningful life experience. I want to touch them again and again.

My Heart Aches for Her

My Ruby is so quiet and tentative at times. Apprehensive may be too strong a word at this stage. She used to be terribly fearful. She now will stand behind the door in the bedroom for many minutes. She is awake, alert as if expecting something or someone. When I find her like this and take her in my arms and tell her I love her, she seems relieved that the spell of waiting has been broken. At times like that, my heart overwhelms me with an aching love for her. Where in the world has the Ruby that I knew gone? This disease is more devastating than death, for it leaves behind an empty shell.

Things of the Spirit

There seem to be things of the spirit in Ruby that are far ahead of me. We who are unafflicted by this disease are so encased by daily occurrences and circumstances that our awareness of our environment puts a shield around us that keeps us from understanding fully the great things of the spirit. It seems to me at times that Ruby has pierced through that and is understanding the deeper things of the spirit that someday we all will comprehend more fully. In some ways she is ahead of me into the world that is to be.

An Outside Latch

Today, I devised an outside latch so that Ruby could not leave the house without our notice. She just gets restless and does not know this is her home. Her spirit longs for "home," and this is not it, even though we own it and have been here nearly five years. Our children's pictures are on the walls, and our names are on the deed, which I have shown her several times. There is a blessed homeland

44

of the soul for which she yearns. When things of earth fade away, the things of heaven become more real.

What a Godsend Irene Is

Two weeks ago, Irene came to stay at our house. She knows how to do the things that need to be done. She doesn't mind driving our car and taking Ruby shopping with her. She is an angel of mercy sent from God. The other night when I came in from a meeting, she was kneeling by Ruby's bed in prayer. The day had not been easy for her, and she was committing it all to God.

I Can't Find it!

Ruby is moving very slowly now. It is difficult for her to get in and out of the car. The other day as I was helping her out, I suggested she give me her hand. She looked all around and said, "I can't find it." But there are bright spots too. Sometimes when she joins me in singing a chorus, she will get every word right. Others have noticed this about her in church. While she cannot find the page number, she will know every word of a hymn.

What Time Is It?

I was resting on the divan the other day where I could not see the face of the grandfather clock. I said to her, "Honey, can you give me the time?" She looked all around, even though she wears a wristwatch. Then I said to her, "You can tell the time by the grandfather clock." She went to the corner and looked all around the base of the clock. "Honey, you will have to look at the face of the clock where the hands are." Finally, she looked high enough to see the face where the hands are and said, "There aren't any hands on it."

Beyond Being a Stranger

For a long time she did not know me. Apparently she

had regressed into teen years, and we did not meet until we were nearly 20 years of age. So I was a stranger in the house. Now she is more and more recognizing me as a person who really cares for her. She welcomes me when I have been gone for an hour or two. When I call for her at day care, where I take her once a week for six hours, she will be waiting for me. When she sees me, her whole face lights up. Her arms reach out to me. It is amazing what is going on inside of her.

On Hands and Knees

I took a little nap the other day, and when I woke up, she was on her hands and knees in front of the fireplace with her head on the carpet. I said to her, "Honey, did you fall?" "No, I'm just praying." There is something of the spirit in her that is active and alive. She seems to sense and see things that elude me, although the obvious she cannot manage at all.

More Ruby Ministries

For half an hour, Dr. Richard Peppard, of the Alzheimer's Research Center, and I had been on the "Encounter" program of radio station CJOR, Vancouver, B.C. Many calls came in. The emcee seemed to be surprised not only at the depth of Ruby's helplessness but also that I was not pulling out my hair over the situation, as he put it. I was able to tell him it was by the grace of God. God is the Potter; we are the clay. I believe deeply that God is making a purpose out of it all. Afterward, he asked me again about my coping ability. He seemed to draw strength from me for his own home situation. When we decided to go public with our affliction, it was to help others in their pain, sorrow, and frustrations. It is happening.

· 11 ·

Love Never Fails

Our love and faith may falter and sometimes do. But when faith and love are held steady, hope always generates in the human spirit. When I put my arms around her and tell her I love her, her spirit seems to comprehend that, even though she is incapable of any human response. It is the riches of faith, love, and hope held steady.

Aloneness

When we are together, then I am the most alone. This is a strange paradox. Especially is this true toward evening. Caregivers call this the "sundowner syndrome." Conversation or communication is a two-way street. This is impossible for her. Her attempts at conversation are often in the form of "Why?" "Why are we here together?" "Why don't we eat dinner?" (when we just did); etc. That is a terrible loneliness. One day I said to her with some sharpness, "Please come sit in this chair so that I can push you to the table." After a bit she said, "Why did you speak to me so sharply?" Out of this darkness that has enveloped her mind, there are still areas of great sensitivity.

Memory Loss Is Not the Worst

If this disease only caused memory loss, it would be easier to understand. This disease destroys reasoning abilities. Nothing makes sense anymore. The simplest instructions are incomprehensible. For instance, "Honey, would you put these two plates on the table?" That totally baffles her. She can't move her thought from the kitchen counter to the table, which is within arm's length. The other day I tried domino blocks, spilling them out on the table. "Let's make some patterns out of these blocks. Let's make a long row here and some squares over there." That was beyond her.

Shaking Motions

Her hands are beginning to make uncontrollable shaking motions at times. When I take hold of her hand, this generally subsides. Often her hands are either hot or cold. Perhaps I should research this aspect a little more and document her state of mind in these changes. I'm told these uncontrollable motions may also affect the face, so that a person is ceaselessly chewing. That would be embarrassing in public.

She Seriously Ran Away

Last Sunday we went to church together and then went out to dinner. On coming home, I sat down in the easy chair, not planning to take a nap, but I did. When I awoke, she was gone. I assumed she had gone to some of the neighbors nearby, and I would be getting a phone call shortly. The phone didn't ring. Also it was intermittently raining. After a while one of the neighbors, out for a Sunday drive, pulled into my driveway. Ruby was with them in the car. They had picked her up on the highway, about half a mile from the house. She very trustingly got into their car, though she did not know them. That is one of the problems with lostness. Anyone could have picked her up. And, of course, had they not known her, what would they have done with her? For months she has not worn the I.D. bracelet I bought for her. She doesn't like it. She seemed glad to see me, but with no apology for having run away.

I Was Praying for You

In the middle of the night I sensed she was gone from her side of the bed. I found her kneeling by my side of the bed. "Honey, what are you doing over here?" She said, "I was praying for you." Who can know the depth of her spirit? The Lord God probably hears her more quickly than He does me. I pray out of my mind, as well as my heart. She prays out of her heart.

Prayer Lifts Life

For weeks now, I have been getting up at 6 A.M. to spend an hour in prayer. It is not always easy, but I like what it does for my life. In that sense, I enjoy it. I am moving through discipline to discovery and then delight.

"I Can't Do Anything Right"

In complete frustration she said, "I can't do anything right," when she was trying to get into bed. The moments of awareness of her own inabilities are the hardest for me to bear. In those moments, she is the most aware of her former efficient, caring, and managing self. It is more acute because she had a tendency to be a perfectionist in nature. She wanted things done right. Now to hear her say, "I can't do anything right," is a terrible burden.

Today Was a Good Day

She smiled more today. We played with a big soft ball, and she was able to throw it back with a good deal of coordination. That was better than when we started this exercise last week. She greeted people at church with a smiling face, even though her words did not always make sense. Maybe she is being healed! *O God, may it be. May it be!* My faith reaches up falteringly.

Quality, Not Quantity

I have neglected my diary for several weeks. Ruby has

been going downhill. She weighs 95 pounds now. Her movements are slow. She has difficulty getting up. A dear friend of mine, who attends my Alzheimer's support group, which I started in Ruby's name, came by to say he had taken his wife, Agnes, to the Menno Hospital. Going to the hospital probably signals nearing the end. I'll be facing that with Ruby, I suppose, before too long.

MSA Manor

By providence, in a restaurant, I met a man by the name of Mr. Ernst Martins. He is the administrator in the MSA Manor, where I gave two programs recently. We had a most interesting conversation. We talked about the 65-bed Alzheimer's unit being built there, where they will develop a program of long-term care for its victims. I posed this question: "To what purpose is this therapy program for these people when there is no hope of a cure at the present time?" He answered me forthrightly, having posed that very question to his governing board. "Our purpose is to give quality care without much regard as to whether that extends the quantity of life remaining. Quality care is our objective—to maximize life while it remains." That expressed my own commitment to Ruby: quality care. When I can no longer give that in our home, with outside help, I will have to put her in long-term care.

Jack

Quite by chance, or better, providence, I met Jack some months ago. He is 66 years old, well-read, and never married. He has become a strong proponent of causes that lean toward the right wing. He is suspicious of governmental leaders and also sometimes suspicious of church leaders. He is a committed Christian and knows he belongs to the Body of Christ, but he is of no particular denomination.

He recounted to me three or four instances where the Lord had used him mightily in praying for the sick. One involved his little niece who had epilepsy. While they were visiting in the room, he began to have a strong feeling of compassion for her and the family. He did nothing about it. In a short time the feeling returned, almost bringing him to tears. Again he did nothing about it, wanting to test the spirit (1 John 4:1). He covenanted then that if it came the third time, he would do whatever came to his mind to do at the time. In a short while he was again overcome with this compassion, and this time he sobbed out to God a prayer for her healing. In a bit, as he looked around, all in the house were crying also with compassion. He then and there laid hands on the little girl and pronounced her healing. That little girl has never had another seizure and is today the mother of two fine children. He does not try to explain it; he just recounts it.

He gave me two or three instances where similar events had happened to him, always with a great sense of compassion. Before separating that day, we joined hands and prayed together to see what God has in mind for Ruby. That is where we left it. That is where it is now—in God's hands.

Dreadful Day

It happened at last. Ruby broke her hip. When I got home, after being gone about an hour, she was still on the floor by her bed upstairs. This happened downstairs, and Irene had managed somehow to get her upstairs but then couldn't get her any farther. It was a strenuous and frightening ordeal for Irene, and she is suffering some back strain. We endured the rest of the day and night, not knowing the depth of her problem. Friday morning, we called the ambulance and took her to emergency. The X ray disclosed that her hip was shattered. Apparently she had fractured it 10 days ago when she fell out in the yard. It finished breaking here in the house.

Choices

At first, doctors told me we had three choices: (1) try to pin it; (2) do major surgery with complete hip replacement; or (3) leave it as it is because of her mental condition. Later, the surgeon said we had only two choices. The pin idea would not work. It was either major surgery or leave it. As we talked about it, there really was no choice. To leave it was to condemn her to constant pain. On the other hand, the surgery is commonplace now. This skilled surgeon said he could do it in 35-40 minutes, and they would start her walking under therapy on the fourth day. As he said, "Her mind may be slipping away, but her body is still here, and we must do the best for her body." Good advice. That goes with my recent conversation with Administrator Ernst Martins about quality care.

Under the Knife

Surgery is always a terribly lonely experience, both for the patient and the loved ones. Ruby just disappeared through those doors, and I was alone.

A complete hip replacement was ordered. The skilled surgeon had told me the operation would not take over 40 minutes. I hadn't counted on the long recovery time. She still had not returned from surgery four hours later. In fact, I finally went home. There was simply nothing I could do.

Recovery

Ruby recovered rapidly from the surgery. On the fourth day, they had her standing up and attempting some steps with support. I tried to explain what had happened and what had been done for her, but she didn't grasp it. She seems to have no awareness of having had surgery.

Otherwise, there are some bright spots. We had our 47th wedding anniversary in the hospital room with flowers, cards from family and friends, and pictures. Irene was with us and took the pictures to share with family. I also made an audiotape of messages as I read cards to her. How much she comprehended, I do not know.

Moments of Brightness

Sometimes when friends come in whom she has not seen for a while, she will brighten and smile at them and say, "I'm glad to see you." This tends to become a bit of a problem, for they see her as better than she is. These friends could well think I am premature in considering long-term care for her. That bothers me.

Dr. Sabir Was Blunt

Dr. Sabir said, "You cannot give Ruby the care she needs now." Later on when I talked to Dr. Bootsman, she confirmed that opinion. I teased her a bit by saying, "But you don't know how good a caregiver I am." Then she outlined a course of action by saying, "We can keep her here in activation ward until there is an opening in long-term care." So the decision was taken somewhat out of my hands. However, in my head I agree, though my heart hurts.

The Activation Ward

The head nurse, Larry Whyte, walked me through the ward today and explained the various procedures and equipment. They have a common dining room, small and cheerful, that will accommodate 20 people. That seems to be the limit on the ward. Their object is to get these patients on to their next destination. That may mean back to their homes or on to long-term care.

Finances

I thank God every day for this Canadian system. Ruby and I pay $440 a year premium. This covers everything. I asked at the desk to settle and was told there are no charges.

They used to charge a small daily user fee, but they dropped that. Personally, I believe in user fees. It helps prevent overuse.

Ruby's Ministries Continue

Sometimes I become aware that ministry is resulting from her suffering. Yesterday, I went across the hall to visit a lady named Betty, who knew Ruby from our church contact. As I spoke words of comfort to this person dying of cancer, I keenly felt Ruby's presence by my side, and so did Betty. As I prayed with her, there were tears of relief and comfort.

Activation Unit

Here they will begin to walk her and put regular house clothes on her. So far they have nothing they can do with her moving hands. She plucks at her bedclothes by the hour. She seems to recognize me when I come into the room, but she soon chooses to ignore me.

Inertia

Inertia creeps at me from the edges. It would be easy to give in to it. Already this house seems too big for me. However, I thank God for it. What a blessing it has been to be here as a part of this caring community and a part of the British Columbia health system. I marvel at it.

Daily Schedule

Every day as I close my prayer time, I make a schedule for the day. This keeps me purposeful and moving forward. There is always room for providential interruptions.

· 12 ·

Father, Let Her Go

With tears of gratitude, I surrender my Ruby to the future and to God. About a week ago, the ladies' prayer group that Ruby had been a part of, and who had been praying earnestly for her healing, were prompted to begin to pray for her safe home-going. They were concerned about what I might think if I heard about it, so I went to them and shared that for the last two weeks I had been led to pray the same way. This greatly relieved their minds. As the scripture says, "There is . . . a time to die" (Eccles. 3:1-2), and Ruby's time is near. So I surrender her with my heart full of love for all the years given us.

The Worst Yet

Last night about ten o'clock the doctor called to say Ruby had fallen out of her chair at the hospital. X rays confirm that the other hip is broken. I could hardly believe it. Today I have communicated through the Spirit with Ruby's spirit. She is heavily sedated and waiting for surgery. When I whispered to her, "I love you deeply and forever," she whispered back that she loved me too.

She is very weak. She must have a complete hip replacement, just 29 days after the other surgery. He showed me the large alloy ball and shank that would be thrust into her upper thigh bone. I went back the second time to Ruby and in my heart bid her good-bye and quoted the 23rd psalm: "Yea, though I walk through the valley of the shadow of death, I will fear no evil" (v. 4). It was amazing how the lines of her face relaxed as I whispered to her.

Undue Life-support Systems

I reminded the doctor that both Ruby and I had signed forms 12 years ago requesting that undue life-support systems not be used on us. Those forms were in our files. He understood and was compassionate. Then he asked me the big question: "If she should die in surgery, do you want us to revive her?" "The answer is no, or the forms we had signed in covenant would be meaningless." "I understand," he said. Then I reminded him of the ancient words, "There is . . . a time to die" and that Ruby's life, by the way we had lived and walked with each other, was complete.

As laypeople, we should understand the doctor's dilemma. In some areas there are even laws that bear on this. These kinds of ethical questions should be discussed with him long before the need arises for a decision. Our firmness will help him agree.

Sudden Tears

Just when I think everything is under control, there is a whelming up in my heart and a sudden splash-over of tears. It surprises me, for I have been generally in control. That does not mean I have not permitted myself to cry, but I always chose to cry over important issues. Now I cry for sheer emotion's sake, and it is good.

The Crucible of Suffering

Suffering is a mystery, but I cannot accept it as meaningless. Ruby's spirit and mine are being refined in this cauldron of suffering. Yesterday for the first time the physiotherapist stood her on her feet. Only once did she utter a little moan of pain, and then they coached her into two little steps. Once when I told her she had broken her other

56

hip, too, she looked at me in surprise and said, "Do you mean that?" She did not want me to leave. It is always difficult, but I have to attend to other things.

What Are *You* Doing with Us?

That question lay almost constantly in my heart. I can see doors of opportunity opening because of Ruby's suffering, but what is the real end of it all? Why could not the spirit fly away to the Divine Maker without this interlude of suffering?

If suffering can be turned into blessing, then why don't we all suffer more and even cheerfully? There are religions and philosophies that torture the body for a supposed benefit to the soul. But that is not the Christian way . . . or is it?

Deep Serenity

The other evening when I went to see Ruby, it seemed her face was crowned, hallowed with deep serenity. It was remarkable. It was angelic. There is something in her spirit that grows stronger and stronger, while mentally she grows weaker. I praise God for that. There are times when we still sing together. How wonderful is the peace of God in such moments. It is deep, central, knowable, and feelable.

Three Kisses

We went through a long period of time, about two years, when Ruby did not know me. We would be in the house together, and she would feel uncomfortable and condemned for being in this house with this strange man. I could not caress her or kiss her cheek, for that would be an affront to her highly tuned Christian conscience. But the other evening, after we had sung our little good-night song, I said to her, "Do you want me to kiss you?" With just a hint of a twinkle in her eye, almost like the Ruby of old, she said, "Three times." What a surprise and pleasure to have her returning mentally, even though she is going down physically. Amazing.

A Low Day

Yesterday was a low day. She was not able to eat or even swallow. I cleansed her mouth with moist swabs. I went from her bedside to the funeral home where some years before we had filed folders with the firm. Ruby and I had always faced the inevitability of death. Years before we had bought side-by-side crypts when we lived in Sacramento, Calif. In the folder was a piece I had written—"I Wouldn't Hold the Sunset Back"—some statistics about us, and the selection of a song or two for the funeral. I checked on the cost of plots, etc. The cost of the funeral will be quite bearable. Attending to these details was a means of leading me back to reality.

· 13 ·

What Is Better than Death?

Being ready for death is better than death itself. At 4 A.M., September 29, 1987, I awakened with a sense of wanting to go to the hospital. I had never done that before. I reasoned with myself, It's rather foolish; she is well cared for. But the urge persisted, and I said to myself, "Well, why not? Has anyone a better right to be by her side than I? Certainly not."

When I walked into her room, she was lying quietly with her eyes open. She held out her thin arms to me and said, "Here comes my husband." After not knowing me for two years, that was an amazing and beautiful surprise. God was already healing her for heaven.

I softly spoke to her of my love and God's love and repeated the Lord's Prayer. As she struggled to respond, I assured her she did not need to. "I know you love me. You have told me that and often demonstrated that through a long lifetime. Just be restful." I kept talking to her and to God.

Everyone who knew us and came under our ministry knew we were a team. Neither of us was complete without the other, and both were completed in each other. Neither one of us had ever known another human being intimately, and I had never, even for a moment, desired another woman. Under my gentle caressing and the murmur of my words, she became very restful and went to sleep.

The Lord gave me this promise from the ancient Word: "It is vain for you to rise up early, to sit up late, to eat the bread of sorrows: for so he giveth his beloved sleep" (Ps. 127:2).

Ah, yes, there comes a time when death is sweeter than life, and so I attend my beloved to give her safe passage.

· 14 ·

Beyond Healing

Every caregiver hopes and prays for a healing. We hope there will be a breakthrough, that there will be answers forthcoming better than what we have today. However, I am at the stage with Ruby where I am beyond asking for her healing. I am asking and believing for her safe and peaceful passage. Great comfort has come to me as I sit by her bedside and occasionally wash her arms and face with a cool, damp cloth. She cannot respond except with a searching gaze from her deep blue eyes that are already seeing things that are invisible. Without any movement of her body, her eyes will suddenly pop open, and I know she is seeing things that are yet to be. In those times, I feel almost like an intruder, except that we have been one flesh over 47 years. For the earthly journey, we were completed in each other, and now she is completed in God just a little ahead of me. I sang to her:

> There is a land that is fairer than day,
>   And by faith we can see it afar;
> For the Father waits over the way,
>   To prepare us a dwelling place there.
> In the sweet by-and-by,
> We shall meet on that beautiful shore.
> —SANFORD F. BENNETT

For those who learn through a lifetime to trust and

61

walk with God, life has a completeness. This is what is being fashioned in Ruby now that she lies in a coma. We call it coma, but her spirit is very actively relating to the new world. What she is now enduring are the birth pangs of the land that is better.

Hearing but Not Responding

I'm convinced now, more than ever, that persons who are in a coma tend to be more aware of their surroundings than it seems to us, even though they cannot respond. Several times when I have gone in to see Ruby these last few days, she has lain there on her side with her eyes open, breathing laboriously. When I whisper to her and remind her of God's nearness, she will close her eyes and appear to be asleep. This tells me she is hearing and that she wants to be off to a better land.

Even the Car Seems Big

We are never prepared for that final separation. Larry, the head nurse, saw me coming down the long hallway. As he approached me, he didn't have to say anything. I knew she was gone. I had sung her to sleep just 10 minutes before she died, and I then had gone to a Canada Prayertime in the mayor's office. At first, I was disappointed at not being there at the moment of death. But on reflection, I can see His way is best. No one can go along on that last journey. Each must go alone. When I drove home from the hospital, suddenly the car, which I had driven many thousands of miles alone, seemed too big for me. Something that belonged was missing.

Because of the dreadful Alzheimer's disease, we have had three years of distancing. But it is still a jolt. The house seems too big. There is an emptiness. Perhaps this is even more noticeable to me because I had her constant care. As I think of it now, in my sorrow, would I choose another path? Not on your life.

God's ways are best ways, I have found it so.
Where'er He leads me, there I will go
And never question when comes the test,
*For I know always, God's ways are best.**

I JUST GO ON . . .

Notes

INTRODUCTION

1. "Coping with Alzheimer's," *Reader's Digest* (December 1986), 125-29.

2. Marguerite Henry Atkins, *Also My Journey: A Personal Story of Alzheimer's* (Wilton, Conn.: Morehouse Barlow Co., 1985), 158.

3. "Coping with Alzheimer's," 125-29.